IMMUNE SYSTEM

101 NATURAL WAYS TO BOOST YOUR IMMUNE SYSTEM, FIGHT GERMS, AND LIVE A HEALTHY LIFE

INTRODUCTION

I want to thank you and congratulate you for buying the book, "Immune System: 101 Natural Ways to Boost Your Immune System, Fight Germs, and Live a Healthy Life".

This book contains proven steps and strategies on how to boost your immunity. The immune system protects us from the natural world. Or rather, the immune system protects us from the threats from the natural world. This book will help you maintain your immune system in the best shape possible.

If you are a young adult, then the book will teach you to be your own mother. When you were young, your mother most likely protected you and made sure that you ate the right foods in order to grow and stay healthy. But, you are an adult now, and you need to know the best foods to eat for your health. Your mother cannot protect you forever, but you can by making yourself the responsible one.

If you are a new parent, the book will help you to be the best parent you can possibly be. It is important that children use the maximum amount of their energy to grow up. A child's growth while he is sick is almost inexistent as most of the energy in the body goes into fighting the infection. If a child falls sick too often, then his chances of overall development is reduced. Hence, it is important that you protect your child the best way possible. This book will help you understand what is best for your child, and also, what is best for your overall health too.

If you are middle-aged or hitting the grey hair age, then it becomes of further importance that you take care of yourself that much more. Your body is not as energetic as it used to be, but you can keep your body's defense in good shape. It is, therefore, important that you follow some good practices when it comes to keeping your immune system working properly. As you can see from the title, this book provides 101 different tips and ways to achieve a great immune system. You might not like a few, you might hate a few, but there will definitely be a few that you love. So, I am trying to help you by spoiling you with choice, but at the end of the day, your health is in your hands. This book is merely pointing the way in the right direction.

Thanks again for downloading this book, I hope you enjoy it.

TABLE OF CONTENTS

CHAPTER 1 – LET'S START WITH THE BASICS

We will learn about ten great foods available in the amazing natural world which will help us boost our immune systems. There is no need for me to mention that it is important for you to maintain a great immune system; however, let me explain why you need a great immune system. The simplest reason as to why you need to have a great immune system is this: your body is attacked by millions and millions of bacteria and other microbes every day, and therefore, it is of utmost importance that you protect your body from such attacks. The best way to do so is by boosting your body's first and most effective line of defense: the immune system. So, without any further delay, let us learn about ten great foods which will help you maintain your immune system in prime condition.

1.   GARLIC

This shouldn't come as a surprise to most of you. If you believe the movies, garlic is supposed to protect you from vampires. If a food item can protect you from the supernatural, how easy must it be for garlic to protect you from threats of the natural world?

Do not get me wrong, I don't mean to say that you are forever immune to all diseases if you consume garlic! All I mean to say is that there is a simple logic behind the myth of garlic protecting against the supernatural. Research has proven that garlic has proven to be a great antibacterial and antiviral food. It is even proven that garlic helps improve the white blood cell count in your body. Most of us hate the smell, and the strong taste of garlic, but you can mask the smell and the taste by either dicing, or smashing a clove before using it in your cooking. You can incorporate garlic into your meals every day, and there are no side effects of eating garlic.

2.   GRAPEFRUIT

Grapefruits have more benefits than we care to know. Grapefruits are essentially rich in Vitamin C, which is a great immune booster, and helps our bodies react better to external threats. The red in grapes indicate that they are rich in bioflavonoid. Bioflavonoids are some of the most essential phytonutrients needed for your system (Phytonutrients- care to notice how there is a 'fight' in the name itself). You can consume a bowl of grapefruit on a regular basis, or even consume in the form of smoothies, slushes or even as a simple juice.

3.   MUSHROOMS

Mushrooms are essentially fungi, but they do seem to exhibit some great antiviral and antibacterial properties. They are also a rich source of niacin and Vitamin B, which keeps your system secure and safe. Mushrooms are also known to be a great source of selenium and antioxidants. Rest assured that this fungus will help you boost your immune system. You can consume mushrooms on a regular basis. Be advised that there are quite a few deadly mushrooms out in the world, but there is nothing to worry about, as most of you would be buying them from a local store near you, and nobody is planning to murder you, anyway.

4.   VEGETABLES

We will discuss the many amazing vegetables which boost our immune systems in the next chapter. This will give you an idea as to why vegetables are a must in your daily diet. Vegetables are rich in carotenoids. Carotenoids are antioxidants and they help maintain your immune system in good condition. Vegetables are good for you, and that is the reason why your mom always insisted that you finish your veggies when you were younger. Listen to your mom, and eat your veggies every day.

5.   CAULIFLOWER

Cauliflower, broccoli, and sprouts are some of food most hated by kids. Cauliflower has Choline, Glutathione, and Antioxidant vitamins. Choline helps maintain the health of cells in our body and also keeps the gastrointestinal system in check. A good gastrointestinal system means that our body destroys more bacteria than we consume on a daily basis. Glutathione has a high content of antioxidant vitamins that help ward off general illness.

6.   NUTS

Nuts are packed with nutrients. They are, in fact, filled with protein, saturated fat, and some fatty acids such as Omega 3 and Omega 6, and are also rich in antioxidants. This combination of nutrients is a common theme in many foods, and helps you to maintain a great immune system. The best time to consume nuts is before you have your first meal of the day. You can consume a cup of nuts every day, but over-consumption of nuts can cause some weight issues. Stick to just one cup of nuts a day, and you will be doing your immune system a big service.

7.   THE ACAI BERRY

Acai berry is usually considered one of the best foods to help you reduce weight. This super food will help you drop some unwanted weight, and is also rich in antioxidants, which help to keep your immune system in great shape. Acai berries help you to ward off chronic illnesses when consumed on a regular basis. Consuming these berries is just not enough; you need to have a good balanced diet to go along with them, too.

8.   THE EGG YOLK

This has been a very controversial food in recent years. Most people simply ignore the yolk because of the high cholesterol count. You need to understand that with moderation, you can eat an egg yolk on a daily basis. It is usually considered that eating two yolks per day allows you to make use of the positive aspects by outweighing the negative aspects. The egg yolk is rich in minerals such as selenium and zinc, and these minerals help in the proper functioning of your immune system. The egg yolk is also rich in protein.

9.   OYSTERS

Any seafood is considered great for your body. It is usually rich in protein and has almost no fat in it. This makes sea food one of the best foods on our planet. Oysters are rich in the zinc, which helps the immune system function better. The mineral zinc has antibacterial properties and antiviral properties too, and this further helps your body. You need not eat oysters on a regular basis, but make sure that you incorporate them into your diets at least on a weekly basis.

10.   YOGURT

Yogurt has live cultures of bacteria and other microbes. The truth is, not all microbes and bacteria are bad for you. Your intestinal tracts are lined with bacteria, which help in the process of digestion. Yogurt helps maintain the health of the gastrointestinal system, thereby increasing your immunity. Make sure that you consume yogurt on a regular basis, especially probiotic yogurt. You can have two to three servings of yogurt a day, and this is considered good for your health. However, moderation is advised, as yogurt is rich in fats too.

CHAPTER 2 – 10 GREAT NATURAL SUPPLEMENTS

Supplements are usually micro nutrients which are as important to your body as macro nutrients. Macro nutrients are protein, fat, and carbohydrates. These three nutrients are the most essential, and the bare minimum requirement in any diet. But, you need to add a few supplements to your diet which help you boost your immune system. Let us look at some of the best natural supplements available all around us.

1.   VITAMIN D

No vitamin in the world is as extensively studied as Vitamin D. All studies have come to the singular conclusion that Vitamin D helps you to boost your immune system. You can consume up to 5000 to 10000 IU of Vitamin D every day. One IU of vitamin D is equivalent to 0.025 micrograms. I am hoping that all of you can do the math. Vitamin D can be created in your body itself if you are subjected to sunlight on a daily basis. If you have a good level of Vitamin D in your blood, you can ward off almost any infection. If you are living in a cold climate, you can take supplements for vitamin D. If you have an infection such as cold or flu, it is often recommended that you increase the intake of Vitamin D to as much as 50,000 IU until the cold or flu subsides.

2.   OMEGA 3 FATTY ACIDS

Omega 3 fatty acids are extremely important for the proper functioning of the human body. Seafood is a very rich source of Omega 3 fatty acids. It was previously considered that vegetarians usually do not have many choices when it comes to adding Omega 3 to their diets. This was proven wrong by many research studies. There are some great vegetarian foods which are rich in Omega 3, such as Brazil nuts and soy beans. The recommended daily dosage of Omega 3 fatty acids required for you is around 4000 mg. Omega 3 supplements will help you to maintain your immune system by boosting the production and effectiveness of white blood cells. In colder countries, it is recommended that you take a tablespoon of cod liver oil, or any other natural omega fatty acid supplement every day.

3.   PROBIOTICS

The name suggests exactly what they are. Probiotics are the useful bacteria, which help in the proper functioning of your body. It is a proven fact that the most obvious threats to our body come from the gastrointestinal parts. It is important that we keep this system as clean and effective as possible. Probiotics will help you keep your digestive tract in perfect health, and also help in the production of a certain type of white blood cells called the T lymphocytes. The dosage is usually varied depending on the individual. You can consult a dietician to know the exact required dosage for your unique body.

4.   ZINC

We have previously read about the ways that zinc helps our body. Zinc aids in the production of white blood cells, and can help in the protection of our bodies from various infections. A regular dose of 50 mg is enough to keep your body in a great condition. Zinc is known to be effective against respiratory infections. High doses of zinc combined with Vitamin C will help reduce the lead content in our bodies, too. Zinc deficiency is prominent in developed countries such as Canada, and the USA. So, it is often advised that you take zinc supplements to keep your health in check.

5.   ASTRAGALUS

Astragalus is a Chinese herb which helps your immune system tremendously. Although it is not as quick acting as Vitamin D or Omega 3, it is a great supplement to add into your diet. 1000 mg or more of this supplement is recommended for everyone. Astragalus takes up to six to eight weeks to show great results, and hence, it is advised that you do not expect immediate effects

6.   SELENIUM

If you are attentive enough, you might have realized that many foods mentioned in the previous chapters had selenium present in them. Selenium is a mineral which is really important for the production of white blood cells. You can take supplements of selenium on a regular basis. The recommended daily dosage is 200 micrograms. Most dieticians recommend taking supplements of vitamin E along with selenium. These two micro nutrients work together synergistically.

7.   VITAMIN A

I am sure all of you must have gotten advice as to how Vitamin A is good for your eyes. This vitamin is good for your eyes, but it is also good for your immune system. Vitamin A helps in the production of T lymphocytes, and B lymphocytes. Both these white blood cells are extremely important in fighting infections. The recommended daily dosage of Vitamin A is 1000 IU, and one IU of vitamin A is equal to 0.3 micrograms in standard units. Vitamin A is present in significant quantities in most multivitamin supplements.

8.   COLOSTRUM

There is a reason why they say breastfeeding is very important. Any mammalian species, after giving birth, starts secreting milk from mammary glands, from which the name, mammals. The milk produced right after childbirth is especially rich in several antigens and antibodies which help protect the newly born. Colostrum is the milk of a cow, which has recently given birth. In more accurate terms, Colostrum is the milk produced by the cow in the first six hours after giving birth. The number of antigens, antibodies, and growth stimulating enzymes and chemicals in colostrum are numerous, and it makes the perfect supplement to boost your immune system.

9.   VITAMIN C

Vitamin C is available in all citrus fruits, but if you are not a big fan of citrus fruits you can take in regular supplements of Vitamin C. The usual recommended dosage is 1000 mg. Over dosage of Vitamin C leads to Diarrhea, but this can be resolved as soon as you reduce the dosage. Vitamin C has great immune enhancing properties and some good antiviral properties.

10.   ECHINACEA

Echinacea is a well-documented immune booster. There are, however, some biased myths surrounding the length of dosage of Echinacea. It was advised that you shouldn't take dosages of Echinacea for more than two to three weeks at a time, but this was proven to be quite wrong, and you can take regular doses of 1000 mg of Echinacea for years on end. Echinacea was also considered to be bad for people suffering from auto-immune diseases, but even this myth was busted. Echinacea was proven to be rich in hyaluronic acid, which is a great anti-inflammatory, and pain reliever. You can have daily doses of Echinacea to prevent and cure many infections.⏷

CHAPTER 3 – 10 GREAT REASONS FOR PHYSICAL ACTIVITIES AND EXERCISES

It is often said that keeping your body in good shape will help you maintain a good immune system. But, the question is, what sort of exercise is good for you, and when is it good for you? Most of you even question whether you can exercise while you are sick. The answer is simple. Regular exercise is great for your health, but overdoing it to boost your immune system is plain outright stupidity. Here are ten great tips and activities regarding exercises which help you maintain your immune system in pristine condition.

1.   Never overdo your exercise. You must have heard somewhere that exercise boosts your immunity and this shouldn't inspire you to work harder than required. If you are looking to reduce weight, then it is advised that you prefer lifting weights rather than indulging heavily in cardio. If you are having weight issues, then it is also obvious that your immune system will not be performing at the same level as a much fitter person. The most obvious way exercise helps you is by improving your overall fitness.

2.   If you run for 10 to 20 minutes a day, then stick to that regimen. If you are a long distance runner, then keep in mind that running for long distances drastically reduces the white blood cell count in your body. It is often advised that you take other supplements to improve your white blood cell count.

3.   It is often misunderstood when people say that exercise boosts your immune system. You need to understand that exercise doesn't directly affect your immune system, but in reality, it helps you to stay fit and healthy. If you are healthy and fit, then your body will have more energy to fight off any infections that threatens it. There are a few theories as to how exercise helps you to improve your immune system in the following four points.

4.   Whatever the form of exercise you choose; the simplest reaction to it is that your breathing rate increases. If you are into aerobic exercises, even then there will be a slight increase in your breathing rate. It is theorized that this

increase in breathing rate increases the chances of bacteria being present in the lungs and the respiratory tracts. This might directly increase your immunity, but remember that this is only a theory. It might not have been proven, but there is no denying the fact that regular exercise boosts your immune system.

5.   There is another theory which states that exercise increases the blood flow, and this helps in increasing the reach of white blood cells and antigens in your body. It is theorized that with the faster and wider movement of blood, there is a chance that the white blood cells and antigens discover infections that were previously left undetected.

6.   If you have a fever, it is because your body is trying to fight off an infection. Bacteria cease to grow at higher temperatures, and therefore, your immune system simply increases your body temperature. Even when you exercise, your body temperature is slightly increased, and this will help fight off infection. This again is a theory which has not been proven quantitatively as of yet.

7.   Stress and our immune systems are directly related. Cortisol and adrenaline are secreted during high stress and anxiety situations. These chemicals might help us, but if they are continuous and never treated, they inhibit the normal functioning of the body and will have an adverse effect on the immune system. Regular exercise helps reduce the mental stress in our body. Any chemicals left during anxiety are also washed out. Exercise also produces endorphins which produce this general sense of euphoria in your brain. The next time you work out, stop and think about how relaxed and calm you feel even though your body is aching.

8.   There are no good exercises or bad exercises when it comes to boosting your immunity. All exercises are good, as long as you do not overdo them. The most important point of regular exercise is that you keep your body fit and healthy.

9.   There has been much research that shows that people who are 'couch potatoes' generally get sick more often than people who exercise even moderately. If you are an extremely lazy person, then I suggest that you get up from your couch and start an easy fitness regimen.

10.   If you are a parent, then bicycling with your kids a couple of times a week can be a moderate exercise, and as well as a great bonding exercise. You can also go for power walks twenty to thirty minutes every day as part of this moderate exercise regime. If you are young and energetic, then it is suggested that going to gym at least four times a week seriously boosts your immune system. For the older readers, a regular session of golf is a good form of exercise too.

I know you were expecting some easy to do exercises at home in this chapter, but the truth is that there is no scientific proof to show that some exercises are better than others at boosting immunity. So, I have dedicated this chapter to explaining how any decent form of exercise can help you improve your immune system.

CHAPTER 4 – 10 GREAT YOGA POSES TO BOOST IMMUNITY

Yoga is often attributed to spiritualism in the western world. However, these days there has been a serious increase in the clientele of Yoga. You can almost find a yoga center on every street in any major city. Why this sudden shift towards to yoga? The reason is that more and more scientific proof is being found that yoga in fact helps the many different systems in our body, and properly functioning internal systems mean that your immune system is in great shape. Here are some great yoga poses which can help you boost your immune system significantly.

1.   VINYASA ADHO MUKHA SVANASANA

This is a warm-up pose in your daily yoga regimen. It is quite difficult to exactly explain how to do this pose, but you will find many free videos on YouTube. Just type the name of this asana and you will get the details with regards to how to achieve the position. It warms up the entire body, and also stretches and strengthens the various muscles. It helps you improve your immunity by increasing the circulation of blood, and this, in turn helps in the movement of the white blood cells all throughout your body.

2.   BHUJANGASANA

This is a fairly easy asana or pose, to replicate at home. It is also called the cobra pose. The idea is to raise your upper body just like a cobra does. Simply type in the name of this pose in Google to find more information on the asana! There are many benefits of this asana or pose:

i.   This pose improves the flexibility of your spine.

ii.   It improves the circulatory system, which in turn boosts your immune system.

iii.   It helps you to reduce stress. Less stress means less cortisol and adrenaline. The lesser these chemicals are produced in our body, the more efficient the rest of the systems will be.

iv.   It helps you to improve your lung capacity.

3.   DHANURASANA

The pose literally translates to bow-shaped pose. It is quite hard to perfect this position initially, but with regular work, you will be able to master it. This pose mainly focuses on your digestive system and will also help you achieve toned lower abs. I have previously mentioned that seventy percent of all threats to our body come through our gut and hence, a good digestive system is a reflection of a good immune system. The other great benefit of this pose is that it increases the strength of white blood cells, and also increases the circulation of the white blood cells in the body.

4.   SETU BHANDASANA

When translated, this pose means a bridge shaped asana. It is an easy pose to achieve, and you can learn further about it online for free. This yoga pose is a back bend, and concentrates on your thymus, and thereby boosting your immune system directly. It affects the circulatory and the respiratory systems as well. It improves the flexibility of your back, and helps you to correct your body posture. If you sloop a lot, then it is advised that you further look up this asana as it might be really helpful for you to correct your pose.

5.   ARDHA CHAKRASANA

In Sanskrit, Ardha literally means half. Chakra means wheel. The name of the asana is literally translated to half wheel pose. This is a back-bending pose too, and lays emphasis on your circulatory and respiratory systems. This pose also affects your thyroid gland, and stimulates proper functioning of the gland. This amazing pose increases the flow of blood in your body, and helps in the proper functioning of pituitary and thyroid glands. The pose also increases the number and strength of white blood cells, which is the basic entity of the immune system. The position also will increase the strength in your lower abdomen, and also helps you free up your hips.

6.   USTRASANA

The asana literally translates to the camel pose. This asana or pose targets the thyroid glands. It is quite hard to follow the explanation of the pose in words, and it is advised that you search the name of the asana in YouTube. The asana helps improve the respiratory system and also improves the circulatory system. You will find it to be a great stress-reliever too. The asana also concentrates on the organs located in the lower abdomen. It helps you to correct your body posture, and improves the overall wellbeing and health of your body.

7.   VIPARITA KARANI

This is an easy asana to explain and follow. Simply lie flat on your back near a wall. Now try to lift your legs vertically until they are parallel to the wall in front of you. You will realize that this asana has a good impact on your abdomen and your digestive system. Any yoga pose is always controlled by breathing. It is important that you maintain a constant breathing rate throughout. If you have any further doubts about how to achieve the pose; a simple Google search of the name will do. You will increase the circulation of blood to your head, and any upper body organs. This asana also helps in boosting your immunity quite dramatically. You will find a sudden surge in your energy levels and a peaceful state in your mind. This in turn reduces your stress levels, and has a direct effect on your immune system.

8.   SALAMBA SIRSASANA

This is a really hard pose to achieve by yourself! It is advised that you get the help of a yoga guru before you do it yourself. This is a very effective yoga pose with many amazing advantages. The pose is a headstand, and you would be vertical all throughout the asana. The pose increases the overall blood flow in your body. It helps in the proper functioning of pituitary and thyroid glands as well. Like I have mentioned earlier, get help before you even try and master the pose.

9.   KAPALABHATI PRANAYAMA

Pranayama are breathing techniques which help you relax and relieve stress. This technique is simple, really. The technique is defined as rapid inhaling followed by mild exhalations. The pose helps you to detoxify and rid yourself of any harmful chemicals in the body. The need for this posture in the modern day cannot be overstated. With the increasing stress in our daily lives, it only becomes more important that we find ways to reduce stress, and this yoga pose is a very good way to do so. The position also helps in improving the respiratory system and the immune system. It is almost meditative and it helps improve your focus.

10.   BALASANA

This is part of restorative yoga. Balasana literally translates to childlike pose. It is a fairly easy pose to master, and there is quite a lot of free information with regards to how this position can be achieved. This pose will help you improve your digestive system, and also improves the working of organs in the abdomen region. Since, the emphasis is on the abdomens, you can see some physical improvements too. The pose also improves the circulatory, respiratory and immune systems.

I agree that there is not a lot of information on how these poses can be achieved. I apologize for this, as the book is about informing ways of improving your immune system. So, I have provided you with the very best poses to improve your immunity among the millions of yoga poses. With a little search of each name online, you will find information on how to achieve these poses. But, rest assured, these ten poses will help you when it comes to boosting your immune system.

CHAPTER 5 – 10 NATURAL DRINKS TO BOOST IMMUNITY

In this chapter, we will talk about some of the best drinks you can prepare at home that will help you boost your immune system. These are some great drinks which you can serve to guests, and can even use them to cool off on a hot summer day. So, let's move on and learn about these ten amazing drinks.

1.   RISE AND SHINE

Most of us drink water immediately after waking up, and trust me; this is a very good habit. If you are not one to drink water early in the morning, then start now. Actually, you can do much better than plain water by adding two readily available ingredients to it. Squeeze a lemon into a glass of hot water. Now, add a tablespoon of ginger to the drink. Stir well until all the ingredients are properly mixed. I know that there are only two ingredients, but the reason why this drink is so effective is more because of the timing rather than anything else. After a long night's sleep, your stomach is mostly empty. Since the stomach is mostly empty, the antibacterial and antiviral properties in ginger help clean the stomach. The citrus fruit provides Vitamin C and many antioxidants which will wake your body up in its entirety. Try this simple and easy drink on a regular basis; in fact make it a habit to start your day with it.

2.   CHAI

This is the traditional Indian tea. Chai is not so different from the normal tea we all make. The Indian version of tea usually has an additional dosage of spices or herbs which help in increasing the immunity and also increase the general energy levels of the body. The usual spices which are added are cloves, ginger, cinnamon, and sometimes, even pepper. The traditional Indian tea has milk in it, but if you are worried about the carbs in the milk, then you can simply avoid the milk and sugar. Chai is a great way to start your day. Try to replace your usual coffee with chai instead. Caffeine present in coffee can create many dormant issues in our body, so it is better to avoid caffeine altogether.

3. SMOOTHIES

Smoothies are often associated with fat and carbohydrates. Basically, we view smoothies as glorified milkshakes. However, you can use these great drinks to energize yourself during the day with right set of ingredients. I am assuming that all of you know how to make a smoothie, so I am only going to speak about the ingredients that can be used to make a delicious immunity-boosting smoothie. Use low sugar ingredients such as berries, grapes, bananas, and apples. Most of us associate bananas with high sugar, but bananas are loaded with carbohydrates that only produce instant energy, and this energy is rarely stored as fats in the body. You can add supplements to your smoothie such as un-denatured whey. This supplement has proven to provide a protein punch and is also a rich source of Omega 3 fatty acids and antioxidants. You can use chia seeds and flax, both rich in Omega 3 and glutathione. Both these micronutrients boost our immune systems, as we have learned in the previous chapters.

4. THE SUPER C

This is an easy smoothie that you can make at home. We already learned about the ways Vitamin C and astragalus can help in boosting our immune system in the previous chapter titled '10 great natural supplements'. This smoothie basically incorporates both these wonderful ingredients into one amazing drink.

Ingredients:

• Two and a half cups of coconut milk (you can use normal milk too, if you are not worried about the calories)

• 1 packet of acai berry pulp

• Vitamin C powder – 500 mg

• Non-denatured whey powder – 1 scoop

• Astragalus powder – 500 mg

• Half a banana

5. MATCHA

Matcha is regular green tea but with ten times the concentration. It is basically powdered green tea leaves. Matcha contains all the goodness of regular chai. You can consume this drink to rejuvenate yourself and boost your immune system at the same time after a long day's work.

6.   MUSHROOMS

We spoke in the very first chapter about the goodness of mushrooms. You can make a drink of mushrooms too. Simply dry the mushrooms, and make a powder out of it. You can make a drink by adding the powdered mushrooms to hot water. You can have yourself an instant immune boosting drink in a few seconds.

7.   MINERAL RICH DRINKS

There are ways to create these drinks at home, too. But, it is really hard to get your hands on all the incredible ingredients. Instead, try some energy drink powders available in a store near you. While you are buying them, make sure you read the ingredients. Only buy the drinks if they are rich in Vitamin A, C, D, and E, Zinc, Selenium, and other immunity boosting herbs such as ginger.

8.   GREEN JUICES

I agree that these juices look disgusting, smell disgusting, and probably will taste disgusting too. There is a reason why they are even made in the first place. They are great for your digestive system and increase the alkalinity of your system. The more alkaline your system, the fewer will be the germs and bacteria in your body. So, try to get beyond the taste, smell, and looks, and simply finish the green juice because it is so very good for your health.

9.   WINE

This must be a surprise to most of you. There might be a few of you who welcome the sight of this word in a book like this. The truth is, wine is rich in antioxidants, and antioxidants are very good for your immune system. So, do not deny yourself a glass of wine from time to time. However, moderation is required.

10.   HONEY IN WATER/ TEA

What was your grandmother's remedy for colds? I bet it was hot tea with honey, or simply hot water with honey. Honey has great properties to help it to fight off bacteria and other such infection-causing microbes. Honey consumed in any form is good for your health and is also good for your immune system. You can even replace sugar with honey in all your favorite recipes.

CHAPTER 6 – 10 VEGETABLES THAT BOOST IMMUNITY

Green vegetables were one of the most hated foods when we were growing up! The truth is they are really good for our bodies, and it is important that we keep them in our daily diets. Here are ten great vegetables which boost your immune system.

1.   CRUCIFEROUS VEGETABLES

Cruciferous vegetables include broccoli, cauliflower, cabbage, lettuce, kale, red cabbage, and bok choy, to just name a few. These vegetables actually are the best when it comes boosting your immunity. The chemical composition of these incredible vegetables is quite unique. These vegetables are rich in sulfurous compounds, but the human body can convert these sulfurous compounds into isothiocyanates (ITC). These ITCs have been proven to rid our bodies of cancerous cells and have shown immune boosting properties. With such amazing benefits, it was really no wonder that we were all forced to eat these veggies as kids.

2.   ONIONS

Onions come in varied colors and tastes, but the only thing that is common is that they are rich in antioxidants. Antioxidants are extremely important in the proper functioning of the immune system in our bodies. Purple and red onions also contain anthocyanins. The quercetin present in onions helps prevent high blood pressure, and other heart related diseases. Onions are also been proven to help the body fight cancerous cells. It is important that you eat onions as part of daily meals.

3.   TOMATOES

Tomatoes taste good both raw and cooked. I know some of you might instantly be shouting at your screen that tomato is a fruit. I agree that it is a fruit, but we make tomato ketchup and not jam, so to me it is a vegetable. And, the rest of the world treats it so. Tomatoes are rich in lycopene. Lycopene is an extremely potent antioxidant. Lycopene is proven to be highly effective against cancerous cells in our bodies. Beta carotene is another effective antioxidant present in tomatoes and this antioxidant helps boosting the immune system. Tomatoes are also rich in fibers, and do not contain fat.

4.   SWEET POTATOES

Sweet potatoes are often remembered on Thanksgiving and almost instantly forgotten afterwards. Sweet potatoes are far superior to the normal fatty potatoes. Sweet potatoes are purple, and the purple tinge is because of the antioxidant, beta carotene. Beta carotene is converted into Vitamin A by the body which helps boost our immune system. Sweet potatoes are a rich source of beta carotene.

5.   BEETS

Beets are some of the best foods in the world. In truth, any vegetable which is brightly colored is amazing for your body. Beets are dark red. Beets are rich in iron, and also help in the production of white blood cells. Iron is a major component of hemoglobin. Hemoglobin helps the blood carry oxygen and carbon dioxide. Beets help you to carry more oxygen in your blood, and thereby improving the functioning of the organs. Beets are also rich in fibers which are required by your body to maintain a good digestive system.

6.   SPINACH

Spinach is so popular in the world because of a printing error back in the early 1900s. The decimal point was moved one point towards the right. What was supposed to be 1.2gm of iron became 12gm of iron. This was the exact reason why spinach gained so much relevance, and why Popeye the sailor man ate spinach to get strength. All things considered, spinach is still a very rich source of iron, zinc and many other minerals. Spinach is also rich in beta carotene. Spinach also contains Vitamin C, and Vitamin B. Spinach is a rich source of fibers and therefore aids in the process of digestion as well.

7.   ASPARAGUS

Asparagus is in this list because of its amazing ability to flush out the harmful chemicals in the body. Asparagus has great diuretic abilities which help in cleansing the body from the inside. Asparagus contains glutathione, an antioxidant which helps in the prevention of heart diseases. It can be consumed on a daily basis, and because of its low fat content, it can be eaten as sides during any meal of the day.

8.   ARTICHOKE

Artichokes are really good for your liver. If you know anything about the liver, then you must know that liver contains a lot of toxins which need to be removed. Artichoke is rich in a substance called cynarin. Cynarin helps in the detoxification of the body. Artichokes are also a good source of Vitamin B which helps maintain proper functioning of the body and improves the alertness of the mind.

9.   RED BELL PEPPERS

Bell peppers come in colors of green, yellow, and red, but the red bell pepper is far more superior in terms of nutritional quality and immune boosting capabilities. The redness in the bell pepper is due to the substance, beta carotene which, as previously mentioned, is converted into Vitamin A by the body to boost the immune system.

10.   CARROTS

You must get the theme by now. If the vegetables are red or purple or orange in color, they are good for your immunity. Carrots were fed to us, and the reason we were supposed to eat them was because they help improve our eye sight. Carrots are also a rich source of beta carotene. To get the best results from carrots, try and consume them raw.

CHAPTER 7 - 10 ESSENTIAL OILS TO BOOST YOUR IMMUNE SYSTEM

Essential oils are extracted from the bark, fruit, flower, roots or any other part of an edible plant. Essential oils are usually aromatic and are a rich source of nutrients. Here are the ten best essential oils for your immune system.

1.   PEPPERMINT OIL

Peppermint is well known as an ingredient which promotes better digestion in the human body. The oil made of peppermint seems to be the most effective. Peppermint oil helps detoxify the body and also aids in respiratory process. Traditionally, peppermint oil has been used to treat cold, flu, and many other such infections. You can use peppermint oil in smoothies, milkshakes, and many other cooking recipes as well.

2.   MANDARIN OIL

Mandarin oil is very aromatic. It has immense potential as a natural immunity boosting essential oil. Mandarin oil helps improve the functioning of the lymph nodes, thereby directly boosting your immune system. Lymph nodes are at the centre of the immune system and they are known to purify various toxins from the body. Mandarin oil can help in the creation of new blood cells and also aid in the effective circulation of blood.

3.   LAUREL OIL

Laurel oil is historically significant. It was regarded both by the Greeks and Romans as one of nature's greatest gifts to mankind. Laurel oil is laden with antioxidants and it seems to be useful in the prevention and cure of various infections in the body. You can add a few drops of laurel oil in your tea every day or simply add a drop or two in your smoothie.

4.   JUNIPER OIL

Made from the bark, fruit, and even the leaves of juniper tree, this blue colored oil is rich in antioxidants and has amazing diuretic properties. It helps flush out the various toxins from your body. It also has many other medicinal properties. You can consume juniper oil on a regular basis in your everyday tea.

5.   GRAPEFRUIT OIL

We have already discussed the immune boosting properties of grapefruit. It is evident that the more concentrated essential oil of grapefruit makes the list. Grapefruit oil is rich in beta carotene and is a rich source of Vitamin A. You can consume grapefruit oil by adding it in pastries or in your baking.

6.   ROSEMARY OIL

Rosemary oil is very strong, and has great antiseptic properties. It is often not advised to consume rosemary oil if it is too concentrated. You can still use the diluted version in many savory recipes you wish to cook. Rosemary oil adds an incredible flavor when used in cooking. Rosemary oil has great antibacterial, antifungal, and antiviral properties which makes it an exceptional addition in your recipes.

7.   JATAMANSI OIL

This is another popular essential oil with strong antibacterial, antifungal, and viral properties. You can consume this oil directly or use it in the recipe of any savory dish you wish to prepare. This oil has been in use since ancient times in both Chinese and Indian medicines.

8.   WHITE THYME OIL

Thyme oil has a natural property to relieve you of chest congestion and bronchial spasms. Thyme oil is loaded with thymol and carvacrol which help relieve chest congestion and helps you keep bronchial spasms in check. It can be used in many savory dishes, adding a distinct flavor and aroma to the dish in question.

9.   TEA TREE OIL

One of the most extensively used essential oil. Tea tree oil has great antibacterial properties, and can be often used to cure many infections. Tea tree oil can provide relief during cold and flu. It is very effective against all sorts of skin disorders. Tea tree oil is a great immune booster as well. Tea tree oil is usually pretty strong; be advised and never consume the oil directly.

10.   LEMON OIL

Lemons are a great source of Vitamin C, and therefore it should come as no surprise that their essential oil is also a rich source of Vitamin C. Lemon oil is a great disinfectant too. Lemon oil can be added to increase the acidity of a dish instead of vinegar. Lemon oil even has many uses in the beauty industry.

CHAPTER 8 – 10 GREAT HERBS TO BOOST IMMUNITY

Herbs have medicinal properties and have been known to cure many small ailments from time immemorial, although modern doctors discount their benefits. Herbs have been put to use for ages now and they have shown visible results. Most of us believe that it takes years of practice before we can successfully extract medicines from plants. The above statement is true, but only partially. There are many medicines which can be extracted without much effort. Here are ten of the most incredible herbs.

1.   ECHINACEA

This is an herb native to North America and can be used on a day to day basic need. Echinacea is a natural immune system booster. In fact, Echinacea is the most sold medicinal herb in the USA. Echinacea has been proven to be a very effective blood purifier too. It is not hard to grow Echinacea in the comforts of your home, and the ingredients required for you to grow these wonderful herbs are available in all organic health stores.

2.   CHAMOMILE

Almost every one of us has heard of chamomile tea and it is an understatement to say that it is a good beverage. Chamomile tea is proven to have various wonderful benefits including aiding those who suffer from insomnia. Insomnia is a problem of the modern and almost every one of us suffers mildly from it. Chamomile tea is a gentle and effective sleep inducer. It is so gentle that you can give it to your children as well. Chamomile also has anti-infection properties and helps in better digestion. Chamomile tea is also a great stress reliever as it helps remove tension and spasms in your muscles.

3.   LEMON BALM

This is an aromatic herb which can be grown in your house without much effort; however, you should make sure that you do not literally grow it inside your house. Lemon Balm is known to attract bees and this can be a problem if the plant is used as a decorative piece in your home. Lemon balm has many therapeutic effects. It can be used directly or can be made into a tea. It effectively helps you recover from fever or cold by allowing your body to sweat freely. Lemon balm is also known to cure insomnia and anxiety. It can also help relieve tension in your muscles.

4.   PEPPERMINT

Every one of us can identify this herb by its more modern substituent, the peppermint chewing gum. Peppermint is an herb very well known for its taste, but it also has other medicinal benefits. Peppermint aids in your digestion. It is better to chew on a few leaves of peppermint than to use a chewing gum. Peppermint helps our body to cope with diarrhea, indigestion, insomnia, nausea, and even headaches.

5.   SAGE

Sage is proven to be effective against sore throats and even tonsillitis. To make tea out of sage, take one tablespoon of freshly chopped sage leaves (or a teaspoon of dried sage leaves), add it to a cup of boiling hot water and let it rest for ten to fifteen minutes. Gargle with the tea and you will find an immediate relief for your sore throat. Sage oil is a great disinfectant and can help in the proper functioning of the lymph nodes.

6.   THYME

Thyme has a natural property to relieve you of chest congestion and bronchial spasms. Thyme is loaded with thymol and carvacrol, which help relieve chest congestion and help you keep bronchial spasms in check. Make a tea out of it by taking 1 tablespoon of fresh thyme leaves or one 1 teaspoon of dried thyme and adding it to boiling water.

7.   CHAMOMILE

Chamomile tea is one of the more famous herbal teas in the world. The process for making chamomile tea is the same, take a tablespoon of the leaves or a teaspoon of dried leaves and use boiling water. Chamomile helps induce sleep and also can be used to reduce body temperature. You can also extract oils from these plants. The easiest step is to purchase a distiller, which is available for a couple of hundred dollars. You can harvest the oils of almost all the herbs. Chamomile oil helps relieve stomach cramps, colic, and spasms. You can also rub the oil on painful and swollen joints Pea for relief.

8.   CORIANDER

Coriander seeds are used for culinary purposes but they can be consumed directly as they help improve your digestion and have amazing anti-diabetic properties. Coriander is a rich source of iron; it can be used to regulate your problems with Anemia. Coriander is considered a natural cure for a majority of eye diseases including conjunctivitis. You can make a poultice from coriander and it helps you cure many skin diseases such as Eczema, rashes, itchy skin, and inflammation. Coriander has good anti-bacterial properties and can be made into concoction to use on wounds and scars

9.   GINGER

Ginger is a versatile root. It can be consumed fresh and it can also be consumed in dried or powdered form in juices and teas as well. Ginger is known to help in digestion and it is usually considered a good habit to consume ginger right after a meal. Ginger helps improve the health of your heart and helps treat morning sickness, too. Ginger also boosts the immune system and helps prevent diseases such as the flu and cold.

10.   SWEET CICELY

The roots of Sweet Cicely can be consumed fresh and helps treat issues such as cough, flatulence, and even weak stomachs. The roots can be infused into brandy or water and is famous as a potent tonic and stimulant. Sweet Cicely is aromatic in all its parts, so it helps improve body odor and bad breath.

CHAPTER 9 – 10 GREAT FRUITS TO BOOST IMMUNITY

Fruits are nature's goodness packed into a single great entity. All fruits are good for your health. Here is a list of few great fruits which are great for your immune system.

1.   APPLES

Apples are a great source of vitamin A, and therefore earn their place in this much coveted list. You can find many other great benefits of eating apples. They are a rich source of fiber and they have a very low fat content. Apples are ideal in many ways and hence the old saying: an apple a day keeps the doctor away.

2.   PEARS

Pears are another great source of vitamin A. Vitamin A is an extremely important micronutrient when it comes to improving your immune system. Pears can be consumed on a daily basis, and they are also rich in other nutrients. Pears help in the production of white blood cells.

3.   ORANGES

Oranges are a great source of Vitamin C. They are also a great source of beta carotene. Beta carotene is converted into Vitamin A by the body. Vitamin A and Vitamin D are helpful in boosting the immune system as previously discussed in the previous chapters.

4.   STRAWBERRIES

Strawberries are a rich source of both Vitamin A and Vitamin C. Strawberries are also known for their low fat content. They can be consumed on a regular basis in juices, shakes, or by themselves.

5.   WATERMELON

This should not come as surprise to anybody. Watermelon is a great source of Vitamin A, but that is not why it makes this list. Watermelon is 90 percent water and the remaining 10 percent is fiber and contains micronutrients such as Vitamin A and zinc. No wonder this fruit made the cut.

6.   CHERRIES

Cherries are a great source of Vitamin A and are also a great source of antioxidants. Antioxidants play in an important role in the proper maintenance of the human immune system.

7.   PLUMS

Plums are a great source of Vitamin A and are also rich in antioxidants. Plums are known to protect the body from cancerous cells. You can eat plums on a regular basis as they are low In fat.

8.   PINEAPPLE

Pineapple is another great choice of fruit. It is rich in Vitamin C and Vitamin A. It is also rich in minerals such as zinc and iron. You can eat pineapple raw or you can make juices and smoothies out of it.

9.   RASPBERRY, BLUEBERRY, OR ANY BRIGHT COLORED BERRIES

Berries are a rich source of Vitamin A. Many of them are also a rich source of Vitamin C. Berries are on the list because of their low fat content and more importantly because of the high concentration of antioxidants.

10.   DATES

They are almost ideal. They have zero percent fat. They are a good source of Vitamin A, Vitamin C, zinc, calcium, and many other antioxidants. You will find many more great fruits everywhere around you. The truth is all fruits are good. You must consume fruits as often as possible to maintain good health and a strong immune system.

CHAPTER 10 – 11 GOOD TIPS TO REMEMBER EVERYTHING WE LEARNED IN THE BOOK

What is the point of reading a book if you cannot remember what it was about? Here are 11 tips to effectively summarize everything we learned in the book.

1.   NOTHING BEATS A GOOD DIET

This one is self-explanatory, really. You have to eat good food to stay healthy. Remember the old saying, we are what we eat.

2.   SUPPLEMENTS ARE ALWAYS AN OPTION

In colder regions, there is a higher chance of a deficiency of Vitamin D because of the lack of sunlight. This is an example to show that you can choose from the various supplements spoken in this book if you are lacking any nutrients.

3.   EXERCISE IS IMPORTANT REGARDLESS OF IMMUNITY BOOST

A decent daily exercise is a must. If you exercise daily, you are bound to have a great immune system.

4.   THE MYSTICAL YOGA

Do you consider yoga to be spiritual, mystical, or religious? Whatever your view on yoga is, the truth is yoga helps you boost your immunity and there is no denying that fact.

5.   DRINK BETTER

You can find many alternatives to water. Do not replace water for it is vital to your health. Simply add a few more ingredients to your water, such as fruits, to improve your immune system.

6.   THE VEGETABLES WE HATE AS KIDS

I cannot think of a better way to say this, eat all the vegetables your mom made you to eat. They are actually good for your health.

7.   ESSENTIAL OILS

Essential oils are basically concentrated nutrients, and nothing more. They are ten times more effective than the actual fruit, or flower in terms of weight.

8.   HERBS: NATURE'S GIFTS

Herbs are medicinal, aromatic, and add a great flavor to your food. Not all herbs fall into all three categories, but whatever the category is, herbs are natural and are great natural remedies for many health issues.

9.   FRUITS: JUICY AND BOUNTIFUL

Fruits are all the goodness of nature packed in one place. There is no denial of this fact, and therefore consume as many fruits as possible.

10.   BE HAPPY, AND ENJOY YOUR LIFE

This is a general advice. However, it is relevant to the topic at hand. If you are enjoying your life, then you are probably living life stress free. I have spoken extensively about the negative affect stress has on our immune system! Thus, you should try to lead a stress free life.

11.   GO OUT MORE

You cannot stay at home, and then expect to develop a great immune system by eating and exercising well. The human body adapts and grows with different situations. Go out more often, and this will help your body learn better about not only social norms, but also about fighting infections.

THANK YOU

Thank you again for buying this book!

I hope this book was able to help you learn and identify various ways to boost your immune naturally. My hope for you is that as you begin using these methods, your health will increase and you will live a fuller life.

The next step is to choose one of the mentioned ways to boost your immune system and integrate that into your life.

Finally, if you enjoyed this book and received any value from it, then I would like to ask you for a favor, would you be kind enough to leave a review for this book on Amazon? It would be greatly appreciated!

Search "Immune System" on Amazon to find the book and leave a review!

Thank you and good luck!